Moctar Maliki Abdoulaye

# Heart failure: diagnostic and therapeutic approach

**Moctar Maliki Abdoulaye**

# Heart failure: diagnostic and therapeutic approach

**ScienciaScripts**

**Imprint**

Any brand names and product names mentioned in this book are subject to trademark, brand or patent protection and are trademarks or registered trademarks of their respective holders. The use of brand names, product names, common names, trade names, product descriptions etc. even without a particular marking in this work is in no way to be construed to mean that such names may be regarded as unrestricted in respect of trademark and brand protection legislation and could thus be used by anyone.

Cover image: www.ingimage.com

This book is a translation from the original published under ISBN 978-613-8-40656-3.

Publisher:
Sciencia Scripts
is a trademark of
Dodo Books Indian Ocean Ltd. and OmniScriptum S.R.L publishing group

120 High Road, East Finchley, London, N2 9ED, United Kingdom
Str. Armeneasca 28/1, office 1, Chisinau MD-2012, Republic of Moldova, Europe
Printed at: see last page
**ISBN: 978-620-5-98960-9**

# SUMMARY

# INTRODUCTION

In Western countries, heart failure is a major public health problem because of its frequency and consequences in terms of morbidity and mortality and its impact on the healthcare system. [1]

In Africa, cardiovascular diseases occupy an important place among hospitalized patients with a prevalence of about 15% and a mortality rate of 10 to 20%. [2]

Heart failure is the only cardiovascular disease whose incidence and prevalence are increasing due to the aging of the population but also to a better management of heart diseases and in particular of ischemic heart diseases, the main etiology, currently, of heart failure. Despite recent therapeutic progress, heart failure remains a serious disease with a high mortality. [1]

Symptoms of heart failure sometimes occur abruptly, but more often the evolution is progressive, the first manifestations being represented by a limitation of effort tolerance, followed by the appearance of dyspnea for less and less important efforts and fatigue. Many patients are in class III or IV of the NYHA classification when they are first seen. Iterative hospitalizations, important drug treatment, and restrictive hygienic and dietary rules contribute to significantly alter the quality of life of these patients and place a very heavy economic burden on them, their families, and society. [3]

Diagnosis of heart failure must be made early in order to implement effective therapies and combat neurohormonal activation and ventricular remodeling.

The clinical diagnosis of heart failure may be easy when the clinical picture is striking and occurs in an evocative context, but it may be more difficult to make in a patient presenting a frugal or atypical form. In front of a suggestive clinical picture, a certain number of complementary examinations must be requested in order to confirm the existence of a possible cardiopathy, to evaluate the degree of alteration of the systolic function, to evaluate the diastolic function and finally to estimate the severity and the prognosis of the disease. [1]

Among the chronic and disabling somatic pathologies, heart failure is characterized not only by a limitation of autonomy, sometimes major, but also and especially by the anxiety-provoking character of dyspnea and the permanent risk of the occurrence of an acute heart rhythm disorder and sudden death. Taking the best care of the patient with heart failure implies a multidisciplinary approach where psychiatrists and psychologists will play their role in more than one way. The aim is to improve the patient's overall quality of life, to detect possible psychiatric complications, in particular major depression, to take into account the management of emotions in the prevention of ventricular rhythm disorders, and to adapt psychological care to the unparalleled experience of heart transplantation. Finally, the psychological approach of the patient with heart failure appears to be essential, without neglecting the support of the entourage but also of the care teams. **[4]**

The objectives of heart failure treatment are therefore multiple: on the one hand, the treatment must improve the patient's functional comfort and quality of life, in particular by allowing him to increase his tolerance to effort and to reduce the number of acute attacks of the disease and hospitalizations; on the other hand, the treatment must be capable of slowing down the evolution of the underlying cardiac disease, and if possible to prolong the patient's survival, in any case not to shorten it.

The natural history of heart failure patients is marked by numerous hospitalizations secondary to cardiac decompensation. This is why the management of chronic heart failure patients must be multidisciplinary after hospitalization, placing the general practitioner at the center of the care system. The management of heart failure and its numerous decompensations represents an ever-increasing financial burden in industrialized countries, weighing heavily on national economies. It is a major public health problem, in terms of mortality, morbidity and cost, with a considerable economic impact on the health system. **[5]**

To provide the best treatment and optimize the use of health system resources, stratification of all aspects of heart failure is essential.

# DEFINITION

Heart failure is defined as the inability of the heart to provide sufficient circulatory output to meet the metabolic needs of the body and/or where the heart is providing the needs but with abnormally high filling pressures. Heart failure is the outcome of most heart diseases. [6]

The practical definition of heart failure, proposed by the European Society of Cardiology, is based on the following three criteria, of which the first two are essential: [6,7]

-   symptoms of heart failure

-   objective evidence of cardiac dysfunction on echocardiography.

-   in case of doubt, favorable response to treatment of heart failure, usually diuretics.

# EPIDEMIOLOGY

In Western countries, heart failure is the only cardiovascular disease whose incidence and prevalence are increasing because of the aging of the population, but also because of better management of heart disease, particularly ischemic heart disease.

## I. Prevalence

The number of patients with heart failure is constantly increasing in industrialized countries. The aging of the population and the improved management of pathologies such as coronary artery disease and hypertension are the main reasons for this.

The prevalence of heart failure depends on the definition applied, but represents about 1-2% of the adult population in developed countries, increasing to >10% in people aged 70 years [8]. The prevalence of heart failure increases rapidly with age from 45 years onwards. In Europe there are at least 15 million patients with heart failure [9, 10, 11, 12, 13].

Menta's study performed in the cardiology department of the Point Hospital <<G>> showed that it was a pathology of the elderly subject with a clear male predominance. [14].

In a study carried out in the cardiology department of the National Hospital of Niamey (Niger), the prevalence of insufficiency was estimated at 35.15% [15]. [15].

The prevalence of heart failure increases rapidly with age starting at 45 years. The average age of heart failure patients is 55.05 years, with extremes from 17 to 96 years. The most affected age group concerns patients over 65 years (34.95%) with a predominance of the male sex (25.24%). [15].

Heart failure is a growing public health problem in the United States. There are approximately 5 million Americans with heart failure, and more than 550,000 new cases are diagnosed each year [16, 17]. The number of heart failure patients could reach 10 million by 2037 with considerable impact on the US healthcare system and represent a significant economic burden [18]. In the Framingham study, the prevalence is in the range of 3‰ to 20‰ [19].

However, this prevalence increases sharply with age: while it is less than 15.53% in subjects aged 45-54 years and 20.38% in subjects aged 55-64 years, it rises to 34.96% in those over 65 years [15].

**Table I:** Distribution by age group in year and by gender. [15]

| Age range | Male | eminin | Total | Percentage |
|-----------|------|--------|-------|------------|
| 16-24 | " | 6 | 6 | 5,82 |
| 25-34 | 7 | 8 | 15 | 14,56 |
| 35-44 | 1 | 6 | 7 | 6,96 |
| 45-54 | 8 | 8 | 16 | 15,53 |
| 55-64 | 17 | 4 | 21 | 20,38 |
| > 65 | 26 | 1 | 36 | 34,96 |

Despite increasing age-adjusted mortality from heart failure, the number of subjects with heart failure is growing. [20, 21]

## II. Incidence

The crude incidence, i.e. without adjustment for age in the general population, varies from 1‰ to 5‰ per year. It increases sharply with age, by 40% per year for subjects over 75 years of age. [22]

In the Framingham study, the average annual incidence was 3‰ in men aged 35-64 years, rising to 10‰ in men aged 65-94 years. The figures were 2‰ and 8‰ for women, respectively. The age-adjusted annual incidence was lower in women than in men under 75 years of age; in the age group above 75 years. [21]

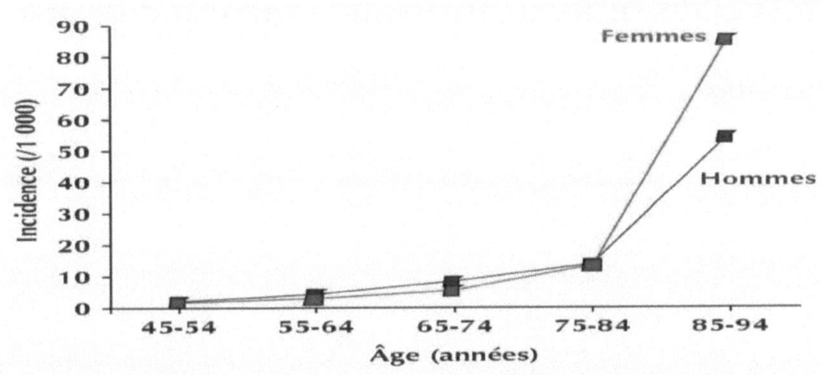


*Figure #1: Annual incidence of heart failure in the Framingham study. [21]*

Based on data from the National Heart, Lung, and Blood Institute:[23, 24]

-the incidence of heart failure increases by 10%o after age 65.

-75% of heart failure patients have a history of high blood pressure.

The most common etiology being coronary artery disease. [25]

In France, the incidence of heart failure is estimated to be between 500,000 and 1 million per year, and 50% of deaths at 5 years in the Framingham study, and almost 50% of deaths at 6 months in patients in class IV of the NYHA. [5]

Its socio-economic impact is major due to the important functional limitation it imposes on patients and the cost of treatment. [6]

# DETERMINANTS OF HEALTHY HEART PERFORMANCE: [26]

**Heart Rate (HR)**

## I. Definition

- DC = Q = F X VES

- F = heart rate;

- SEV = systolic ejection volume;

- Q = cardiac output (expressed in l/min)

- Cardiac index = Q/SC (l/min/m2)

- SC = body surface area;

- The normal cardiac index is between 3 and 3.5 l/min/m2.

- Thus, cardiac output can vary with heart rate and/or stroke volume.

## II. Heart rate

- At rest, in healthy subjects, heart rate has little effect on cardiac output.

- During exercise, tachycardia is the most important adaptation mechanism.

- Tachycardia is also an adaptive mechanism in heart failure (7).

## III. Systolic ejection volume (SEV) [6]

The SEV of the ventricle is determined by three factors: preload, myocardial contractility, and afterload.

- **Preload: length of the muscle at the start of the contraction**

It is represented by the volume of blood contained in the ventricle at the end of diastole. Several parameters influence it:

- total blood mass: hemorrhage or dehydration decrease total blood mass and preload resulting in decreased ventricular performance.

- total blood mass distribution: preload is influenced by the ratio of the intrathoracic to the extrathoracic portion of the total volume; several elements modify this ratio:

- the position of the body

- intrathoracic pressure

- intrapericardial pressure

- venous return

- atrial contraction: increases ventricular filling and volume

telediastolic pressure; its disappearance (in case of atrial fibrillation) or its desynchronization (atrioventricular block) leads to a decrease in ventricular volume and telediastolic pressure

- **Myocardial contraction: the inotropic state** is influenced by the following:

- the sympathetic system, releasing noradrenaline, activates on the receptors

beta-adrenergic ;

- circulating catecholamine levels;

- physiological depressants: hypoxia, hypercapnia, acidosis;

- ventricular mass: a temporary amputation (transient ischemia) or

of a part of the muscle mass leads to a proportional decrease in the efficiency of the affected ventricle;

- Intrinsic contractile capacity: may be impaired, thereby lowering ventricular performance.

- **Afterload:** can be defined as the tension that develops in the ventricular wall during ejection. The degree of muscle fiber shortening determines the stroke volume.

## PATHOPHYSIOLOGY OF IC: [6, 26, 27, 28, 29, 30, 31, 32]

Heart failure (HF) is usually defined as an **inability of** the heart **to provide** with normal filling pressures <<i.e., neither lowered by hypovolemia nor increased >>, **a systemic flow** necessary for the body's need, both at rest and during exercise. In the majority of cases, this heart failure is the consequence of an inability of the heart to empty itself properly by an abnormality of inotropism and / or modification of the afterload. These failures by alteration of the systolic function are the most classical and best known. Another form of heart failure tends to increase in prevalence because of changes in etiological profiles and especially because of the aging of the population: diastolic heart failure.

The pathophysiology of heart failure is very complex.

Some data are acquired:

- hemodynamic alterations largely precede the clinical picture;

- the essential phenomenon is a reduction in myocardial contractile capacity, primary or secondary to extreme barometric or volumetric overload.

Currently, it is considered that the manifestations of heart failure appear not as a reflection of anatomical damage to the heart, but of compensatory mechanisms, hemodynamic and neuro-hormonal, overwhelmed or exhausted.

## I. Compensating mechanisms:

Heart failure develops when myocardial cell function falls below a critical threshold. This leads to stimulation of the neuro-hormonal and hemodynamic systems, in order to increase the contractile force of the myocardium and thus preserve cardiac function.

- Hemodynamic response: a decrease in the capacity to empty the ventricle during systole increases the parietal tension of the healthy myocardium during diastole; the ventricle responds to this increase in parietal tension by increasing the power of the contractions (Frank-Starling law);

- Neurohormonal response: a decrease in the capacity of the ventricle to eject blood activates the sympathetic nervous system; stimulation of beta-adrenergic receptors in the healthy myocardium leads to an increase in the strength and frequency of contractions.

These hemodynamic and neuro-hormonal mechanisms supporting inotropic failure of the heart introduce an important risk: the alteration of the cardiac architecture and the acceleration of energy expenditure. To prevent such functional and structural effects, there is a regulation of the amplitude of the ventricular dilatation and the activation of the sympathetic nervous system:

- **at the ventricular level**: the increase in parietal thickness reduces ventricular tension and dilation; cardiac hypertrophy therefore reduces the energy expenditure of the heart;

- **at the atrial level**: the increase in diastolic parietal pressure suppresses the actions of the sympathetic nervous system; atrial stretch stimulates atrial baroreceptors, which cause the secretion of peptic natriuretic factor (NP), which inhibits the release of norepinephrine and its action on peripheral blood vessels; NP also exerts vasodilatory and natriuretic effects that reduce the hemodynamic load of the heart.

**II. Loss of compensatory mechanisms:**

**1. Loss of parietal tension reduction mechanisms**

Prolonged ventricular distension leads to thinning, necrosis, and then fibrosis of the ventricular wall, which compromises the hypertrophic response and decreases the ability of the heart to normalize parietal pressure.

Prolonged atrial distension leads to structural and functional modification of the atrial receptor resulting in a decreased ability of the receptors to inhibit sympathetic discharge from the vasomotor center.

The consequences are progression of ventricular dilation and permanent activation of the sympathetic nervous system. Heart failure begins.

## 2.   Loss of positive inotropic mechanisms

In the long term, continuously stimulated inotropic mechanisms lose their effects on myocardial contractility.

The failing heart loses power:

-   increase its inotropism in response to an increase in volume

ventricular (preload)

-   to respond to the positive inotropic effects of endogenous and exogenous catecholamines;

-   to increase its contractile function to overcome the increase in

resistance (afterload), the heart is less able to contract and must use this limited capacity to overcome tension rather than to eject blood. Systolic function cannot be maintained, cardiac output drops.

## 3.   Consequences of sustained neurohormonal activation

When cardiac output decreases, systemic perfusion pressure is maintained by two mechanisms: peripheral vasoconstriction and sodium retention.

## III.  Pathophysiological classifications of heart failure: [6]

## 1.   Depending on the dysfunction:

**Systolic dysfunction**

In so-called systolic heart failure, it is the decrease in inotropism, i.e. contractility, which decreases ventricular performance by lowering the systolic ejection volume, with alteration of ventricular filling, and cavitary dilatation. The typical example is primary dilated cardiomyopathy.

**Diastolic dysfunction**

It is the ventricular relaxation that is abnormal.

**Systolo-diastolic dysfunction**

-Very often, hypertrophy and dilatation are associated. The ventricle fills and contracts abnormally.

**2.    Depending on the cardiac output**

**Heart failure with decreased or increased cardiac output**

Some diseases are accompanied by an increase in cardiac output and lead in their evolutionary course to the appearance of heart failure. Anemia, hyperthyroidism, arteriovenous fistula, Paget's disease and beriberi constitute the main diseases of a hyperflow. The heart is forced to circulate an abnormal amount of blood.

In the vast majority of cases, there is a decrease in cardiac output.

**3.    Hemodynamic forms**

Heart failure occurs as a result of mechanical overload of the heart pump.

**Mechanical overload:**

**>    Volumetric overload**

It is the consequence of an increase in ventricular end-diastolic volume. The ventricle must eject an abnormally large amount of blood at each systole to maintain sufficient systemic flow. The ventricle dilates. This is the case of regurgitating valvulopathies (mitral, aortic, tricuspid insufficiency), or shunts;

**>    Barometric overload**

It is the consequence of an increase in afterload by elevation of systemic pressures (arterial hypertension) and/or obstacle to ventricular emptying (aortic or pulmonary narrowing) which leads to ventricular hypertrophy.

**4.    According to the evolution: acute and chronic heart failure**

Myocardial infarction and sudden valve leakage are the cause of acute heart failure, in which the clinical situation is immediately worrying and dominated by dyspnea and arterial hypotension.

On the other hand, a progressive deterioration of the cardiac function leads to the appearance of peripheral signs, spread out over a more or less long period.

## 5.   Depending on the cavities affected: right and left heart failure

The compensation mechanisms can be exceeded, either because of the evolution of the cardiopathy, or because of additional factors. Heart failure is then said to be decompensated. Clinical signs appear, linked to :

- **at the level of the failing ventricle**, the amount of blood ejected decreases, hence:

- increased ventricular end-diastolic volume;

- increased pressure with decreased ventricular ejection fraction.

- **downstream of the failing ventricle**:

- lowered ventricular output

- peripheral hypoperfusion (of noble organs)

- **upstream of the ventricle fail**:

- increased telediastolic pressure, venous stasis, increased capillary pressure: it is this increase in pressure that explains the peripheral signs.

### *S* Left ventricular failure

Upstream of the left ventricle, pressures rise in the left atrium, then in the pulmonary capillaries, causing acute pulmonary oedema (APO), which triggers coughing. Downstream of the left ventricle, the reduction in cardiac output initially leads to a redistribution of local circulation to the benefit of the heart and brain, to the detriment of the muscular, cutaneous, splanchnic, and renal territories. At a more advanced stage, the decrease in cardiac output results in asthenia. At the end of the evolution, cerebral hypoperfusion can lead to confusion, agitation or obnubilation.

### *S* Right ventricular failure

Venous hyperpressure affects the vena cava territory and explains :

- turgidity of the jugular veins (TVJ).

- hepatomegaly (heart liver)

- hepato-jugular reflux (HJR)

- ascites

- edema of the lower limbs (IMO), bursa in men, labia majora in women, abdominal walls leading to anasarca.

The combination of venous hyperpressure and decreased cardiac output results in the alteration of the following functions:

- renal: hydro sodium retention, responsible for oedemas, serous effusions, and weight gain;

- hepatic: increase in bilirubin and transaminases in the blood, followed by a drop in the prothrombin level;

- cerebral: mental disorders (insomnia, agitation, or on the contrary drowsiness, torpor) and respiratory disorders (Cheyne-Stokes respiration).

# MANIFESTATIONS OF HEART FAILURE

## 1. Left ventricular failure (LVF)

### 1. Clinical signs

**Functional signs:[33]**

- **Dyspnea**

It is the most frequent manifestation of GVI. It is a subjective phenomenon, which each patient describes in a particular way, according to his usual lifestyle and physical activity.

- Typically the onset is progressive: superficial polypnea, triggered by effort, becoming progressively disabling.

- When dyspnea occurs at rest, it is referred to as orthopnea.

- Other aspects of dyspnea are multiple:

- the most classic is the acute pulmonary oedema (OAP): of occurrence

sudden and unexpected, whatever the previous state, sometimes inaugural, characterized by the installation of a superficial polypnea with thirst for air, sensation of thoracic fullness and metaphysical anguish; crackling rales at the pulmonary auscultation

- pseudo cardiac asthma: expiratory bradypnea with diffuse sibilance and viscous sputum.

- It is customary to evaluate the functional gene of the heart according to the New York Heart Association (NYHA) functional classification, which considers four progressive stages.

- **NYHA CLASSIFICATION: [1]**

- **stage I**: patient with asymptomatic heart disease.

- **stage II**: patient bothered by breathlessness or fatigue for important and unusual efforts.

- **stage III**: patient with difficulty in performing everyday activities.

- **stage IV**: patient with effortless dyspnea or dyspnea at rest

Many patients are in NYHA class III or IV when first seen. **[15]**

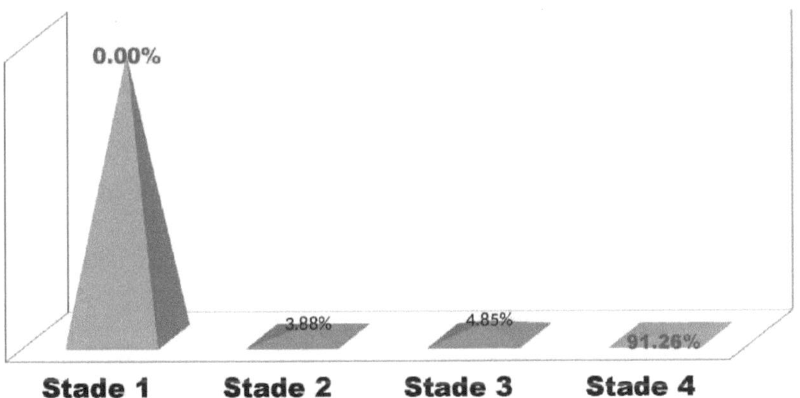


*Figure #2: Percentage of patients by NYHA classification in a prospective study [15].*

- **Coughing**

This is the second basic symptom. The cough is usually dry or with sputum more often mucous than frothy. **[33]**

- **Other functional signs,** are suggestive:

- palpitations may be observed, either in isolation or in fits;

- syncope due to acute circulatory failure

**General signs**

- the general signs found are asthenia, the most frequent observed in 96.12%, anorexia found in 82.52% and weight loss observed in 44.66% **[15]**

**Physical signs**

- Pulse: often rapid (compensatory mechanism that increases cardiac output: (Q=F x VES), often alternating (succession of equidistant beats, one weak and the other more ample)

- Blood pressure (BP): may be low, reflecting a decrease in stroke volume (ESV), or pinched.

- Precordial palpation may detect a leftward and downward deviation of the peak shock and its spreading, indicating enlargement of the left ventricular cavity.

- Cardiac auscultation:

• resting tachycardia, sometimes irregular (tachyarrhythmia)

• the galloping sound, a fundamental sign, heard in protodiastolic position contemporary with the rapid ventricular filling phase (B3), or in the presystolic position contemporary with atrial systole (B4).

• A soft, high frequency, holosystolic, apexo-axillary functional mitral insufficiency murmur, giving a steam jet tone.

• Pulmonary auscultation: is a good reflection of the intensity of the insufficiency left ventricular, all intermediates being possible between normal auscultation and the rising tidal crackles of acute pulmonary edema.

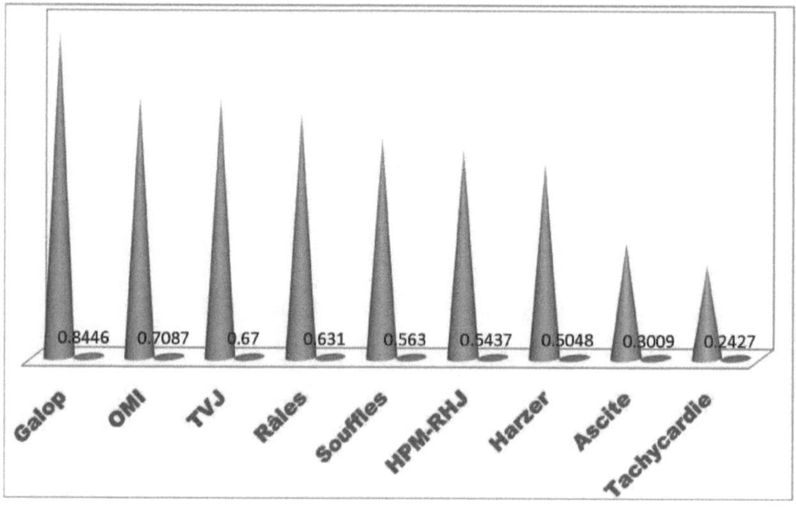


*Figure 3: Prevalence of physical signs in a prospective study [15].*

## 2.  Additional examinations

### 2.1  Chest X-ray

Chest radiography has lost interest since the advent of ultrasound techniques. It allows to appreciate the size of the cardiac silhouette and the pulmonary stasis.

Cardiomegaly can be detected as evidenced by the increased cardiothoracic ratio (normal < 0.50), with in left ventricular dilatation a protrusion of the left inferior arch dipping below the diaphragm; in right ventricular dilatations, however, the tip remains supradiaphragmatic. However, the absence of cardiomegaly does not rule out the diagnosis of heart failure. Cardiomegaly is usually absent in patients with acute heart failure and in cases of diastolic dysfunction;

Pulmonary stasis is manifested in order of increasing severity by:

-    a tendency to vascular redistribution from the base to the tops.

-    interstitial edema with Kerley's lines, and blurred appearance of the large hilar vessels and reticulonodular images predominating at the bases;

-    alveolar edema with flaky opacities with blurred contours extending from the hilum to the periphery (so-called "butterfly wing" appearance), these opacities are most often bilateral but misleading unilateral forms may be seen. [1]

### 2.2  Electrocardiogram (ECG)

It has no value in assessing ventricular function.

It is useful in determining the cause or triggers of an acute attack. We look for:[34]

-    sinus tachycardia or a rhythm disorder, such as complete arrhythmia by atrial fibrillation or atrial flutter;

-    a conduction disorder: high-degree atrioventricular block or complete left bundle branch block which is quite common in primary cardiomyopathies;

-    signs of ischemia or recent or old infarction;

-    signs of left ventricular hypertrophy (Sokolow 35 mV);

- signs of left atrial hypertrophy.

## 2.3 Doppler echocardiography:[34]

Echocardiography is the key examination in the evaluation of heart failure patients. It confirms the diagnosis of heart failure, participates in the etiological investigation and provides prognostic elements.

- **Diagnostically, echocardiography can distinguish:**

- Systolic heart failure: the systolic and diastolic diameters of the left ventricle are increased, the shortening fraction is decreased, as well as the ejection fraction and cardiac output. Transmitral flow measurement shows a decreased diastolic filling time with early filling (E wave), important in functional mitral insufficiency;

- diastolic heart failure: the diameters of the left ventricle are normal or close to normal, the walls of the left ventricle are sometimes thickened, indicating hypertrophy, the measurement of the mitral flow shows a decreased initial E wave with a slowed decay and an increased A wave corresponding to the atrial systole

- High output heart failure with hyperkinetic appearance of the left ventricle, high cardiac output.

It also allows the evaluation of pulmonary pressures.

- **On the etiological level,**

It allows to specify the ischemic origin and to show abnormalities of the segmental kinetics, to look for a valvulopathy by measuring the direction and the speed of the flows in Doppler or a hypertrophic and obstructive cardiopathy by showing a dynamic obstacle to the ejection of the left ventricle.

- **It also allows us to assess the prognosis**

By specifying the extent of ventricular remodeling: hypertrophy or dilatation and to look for intracavitary contrasts or thrombi.

- **Finally it allows a classification** based on the value of the left ventricular ejection fraction (LVEF): **[35]**

## 2.4  Biology: [26]

**Essential examinations in cases of apparently idiopathic abortion, as they diagnose causes that are potentially accessible to treatment:**

- Thyroid workup (TSH, free T4) in search of dysthyroidism

- Martial assessment (ferritin), in search of hemochromatosis.

- CBC: anemia, cause or aggravating factor.

- Search for a vitamin B1 deficiency.

- Calcemia, phosphoremia: hypocalcemia

- HIV serology 1-2 if young subject

**Prognostic and therapeutic follow-up biological examinations:**

- blood and urine analysis (hyponatremia, dyskalemia...).

- Urea, creatinine, GFR: functional renal failure

- Young blood glucose, HbA1c, lipid profile if coronary patient

- Protein and albumin levels: undernutrition, poor prognosis

- Hepatic workup (liver shock in high flow rates).

**Place of Brain Natriuretic Peptide (BNP):**

In response to an increase in volume, thickness or parietal tension, the myocyte can release pro-BNP, NT-proBNP and BNP

Positive diagnosis of dyspnea:

BNP < 100 pg/ml and NT-proBNP < 400 pg/ml: dyspnea of non-cardiac cause, probable pulmonary origin

BNP 100-400 pg/ml and NT-proBNP 400-2000 pg/ml: not very contributory, need for other tests

BNP > 400 pg/mL and Nt-proBNP > 2000 pg/mL: dyspnea of cardiogenic origin very likely.

## 2.5 Other complementary examinations [36]

**Transesophageal echocardiography (TEE)**

Transesophageal echocardiography is not necessary for the diagnostic evaluation of heart failure; however, it may be useful in certain clinical situations such as suspected aortic dissection, infective endocarditis, or congenital heart disease and to exclude intracavitary thrombi in patients with AF requiring cardioversion. When the severity of mitral or aortic valve disease does not match the patient's symptoms on Trans thoracic echocardiography, a TEE examination should be performed.

**Stress echocardiography**

Stress echocardiography, either pharmacological or stress, can be used for the evaluation of inducible ischemia and/or myocardial viability and in patients with valvular disease (e.g., dynamic mitral regurgitation, low-flow, low-gradient aortic stenosis).

**Cardiac magnetic resonance (CMR)**

CMR is recognized as the gold standard for volume, mass, and ejection fraction measurements of both the left and right ventricles. It is the best alternative cardiac imaging modality for patients for whom echocardiography is nondiagnostic (especially for right heart analysis) and is the method of choice in patients with complex congenital heart disease and for the evaluation of myocardial fibrosis. In addition, CMR allows the diagnosis of certainty of myocarditis, cardiac amyloidosis, cardiac sarcoidosis, Chagas disease, ventricular noncompaction, Fabry disease and hemochromatosis.

**Single photon emission computed tomography (SPECT)**

It can be useful in the assessment of ischemia and myocardial viability. Pulsed emission tomography (PET) can also provide information on ventricular volumes and function, but it exposes the patient to ionizing radiation.

**Coronary angiography**

The indications for coronary angiography in patients with heart failure are in accordance with the recommendations of the European Society of Cardiology. Coronary angiography is recommended in patients with heart failure who suffer from angina despite medical treatment. Coronary angiography is also recommended in patients with a history of symptomatic ventricular arrhythmia or recurrent cardiac arrest. Coronary angiography should be considered in patients with heart failure and an intermediate to high pretest probability of coronary artery disease and the presence of ischemia on noninvasive stress tests to establish the ischemic etiology and severity of coronary artery disease.

## 3. Evolution-prognosis of left heart failure:[26]

### 3.1 Evolution

- **Rapidly fatal left heart failure**

- In the acute phase of infarction, myocardial destruction greater than 40% creates irreversible cardiogenic shock.

- During acute myocarditis, the evolution is sometimes superacute; recovery is possible, sometimes complete, but remains unpredictable.

- The use of emergency transplantation is debatable in the young subject.

- **Left heart failure evolves most often by attacks**

- The first decompensation usually evolves favorably.

- Other episodes occur, often with a triggering factor

- The risk is the appearance of permanent and disabling dyspnea

- Progression to congestive heart failure is a poor prognostic turning point.

- **Some complications hasten the progression**

- Supraventricular or ventricular rhythm disorders, with their risk of sudden death, to be detected by repeated Holter.

- Thromboembolic events.

- Iatrogenic complications (diuretics, digitalis, VKA, ACE inhibitors).

- Sudden death is always possible.

## 3.2 Prognosis

- **Mortality**

- Often very high (greater than 50%) at two years for NYHA classes III and IV.

- Appears to be improved by treatment, especially ACE inhibitors and beta-blockers.

- **Clinical factors of poor prognosis**

- NYHA class III or IV.

- B3 (third heart sound).

- Pinched blood pressure (BP).

- Lowered maximal oxygen consumption (VO2) (< 15/ml/kg/min).

- **Hemodynamic factors**

- Lowered EF (<30%).

- LV dilatation.

- **Electrophysiological factors**

- Presence of severe ventricular arrhythmias on Holter.

- **Biological abnormalities of poor prognosis**

- Hyponatremia.

- Renal insufficiency.

- High BNP and no decrease under medical treatment.

- Increase in plasma norepinephrine.

- Increase in atrial natriuretic factor.

## II. Right ventricular failure (RVF):[26]

Right ventricular failure (RVF) is defined as an increase in right ventricular end-diastolic pressure; the right ventricle cannot adapt its output to the peripheral venous return. RVF is most often due to the evolution of a left heart failure (congestive heart failure).

- **. Clinical signs**

**Functional signs**

- **Exercise-induced hepatalgia**

Dull pain, like heaviness, occurring with effort (walking):

- located in the epigastrium or the right hypochondrium.

- giving way a few minutes after the effort it imposes has been stopped.

- it is sometimes associated with digestive disorders.

**Spontaneous hepatalgia**

Occurs during IVD flare-ups, sometimes simulating a digestive emergency or hepatic colic.

- **Permanent late-stage hepatalgia**

Increased during exercise or postprandially with a sensation of distension of the right hypochondrium.

- **Dyspnea,** related to the abortion or to the causative respiratory disease.

**Physical signs**

- **Peripheral level:**

- Jugular venous turgidity present at rest, in a half sitting position.

- diffuse, firm, smooth, painful hepatomegaly, sometimes with systolic expansion corresponding to tricuspid insufficiency; measured on the midclavicular line, the hepatomegaly follows the variations of the IVD (accordion liver).

- Hepato-jugular reflux, which is found in a half-seated subject, breathing normally, after compression of the hepatic region, is the most important sign of cardiac liver.

- Edema is seen at an advanced stage of IVD; sometimes it is detected by a simple weight measurement; elsewhere it is clearly visible: white, soft, painless, and bucket-shaped, it predominates in the lower limbs and, at a later stage, in the lumbar region.

- oliguria: early, with dark, low-sodium urine; functional renal failure

- at an advanced stage of IVD, anasarca: ascites, bilateral pleural effusions (protid-poor transudates).

- cyanosis: it is most often due to the causal respiratory insufficiency and to the obstruction of venous return.

- **Cardiac level:**

- Harzer's sign: palpation of the right ventricle in the epigastric cavity

- on auscultation:

- persistent tachycardia at rest;

- B2 burst at the pulmonary focus in PAH, with ejectional systolic murmur at the pulmonary focus;

- xiphoidal right gallop clearer on inspiration;

- holosystolic murmur of tricuspid insufficiency at the xiphoid level, appearing or increasing with deep inspiration (Carvalho's sign)

-      **Identification of signs of the causative condition**

-      Cardiac or pulmonary, often in the foreground.

## 2.      Complementary examinations in right heart failure

**Electrocardiogram (ECG)**

•      Sinus tachycardia most often.

•      Signs of right atrial hypertrophy: right deviation of the P axis; ample P wave greater than 2.5 mm in D2, D3, VF, and sharp, normal duration.

•      Signs of right ventricular hypertrophy: right deviation of the QRS axis, large R wave in V1, large S wave in V5, left deviated transition zone; frequency of right incomplete block; negative T wave in right precordial.

**Radiology**

It highlights the hypertrophy-dilatation of the right cavities.

•      Front:

•      right inferior arch overhang (dilated DO);

•      raised, rounded, supra-diaphragmatic tip: elongated left inferior arch (dilatation of the VD), hoof-like appearance.

•      Right anterior oblique (RAO) projection of the pulmonary infundibulum.

•      In left anterior oblique (LAO), filling of the retrosternal clear space and protrusion anterior to the right ventricle :

•      in case of pulmonary arterial hypertension (PAH), convex left middle arch and dilated pulmonary artery branches;

It allows to highlight anomalies specific to the etiology (pneumopahy)

**Echocardiogram and cardiac Doppler**

It highlights the dilation of the right ventricle and the paradoxical septum; it often provides information for etiological purposes. Doppler searches for and quantifies tricuspid insufficiency, which allows calculation of the systolic pulmonary artery pressure (PAPs).

**Right catheterization**

It is indicated only when a surgical cure is envisaged.

He found elevated central venous pressure, elevated middle right atrial pressure, elevated right ventricular diastolic pressures, and a drop in the cardiac index.

The level of pulmonary pressures is specified and differentiates pre- and post-capillary PAH.

**Isotopic angiography of the VD: decrease of the VD ejection fraction.**

**3.    Evolution of the DCI**

The evolution is followed on the curves of weight, diuresis, the hepatic balance, the radio and the ECG.

The evolution depends on the etiology

- In the absence of etiological curative treatment, the evolution is progressively unfavorable, sometimes brutally decompensated by a rhythm disorder, an infection (influenza) or a pulmonary embolism or a drug overdose.

**111. Congestive heart failure**

-    This is the outcome of any right or left heart failure that is very

and all cardiac diseases. It associates the signs of IVG and the signs of IVD.

-    Galloping noise (84.46%), lower extremity edema (70.87%), crepitus rales 63.10%, TVJ (67%), HPM + RHJ (54.37%) are the most frequent signs in heart failure patients. **[15]**

# DIAGNOSIS OF HEART FAILURE

## 1. Positive diagnosis:[1]

## 1. Acute or chronic heart failure

Chronic heart failure, often with acute episodes, is the usual form of heart failure. The term acute heart failure is often used exclusively to refer to acute cardiogenic dyspnea with signs of pulmonary congestion or even pulmonary edema, but it can also be applied to cardiogenic shock, which is a syndrome consisting of low blood pressure, oliguria, and cold extremities. In acute heart failure, cardiac damage is so severe and abrupt from the outset that adaptive mechanisms will not have time to develop or will not be sufficiently effective. The usual causes of acute heart failure are massive myocardial infarction, acute myocarditis, rapid tachycardia (>180/min) or extreme bradycardia (<35/min), acute valvular regurgitation (mitral or aortic insufficiency due to endocarditis, mitral insufficiency due to rupture of cord or pillar), tamponade, massive pulmonary embolism...

Chronic heart failure involves a longer and slower course over weeks, months, or even years, during which time the coping mechanisms have time to develop. Patients may remain asymptomatic or paucisymptomatic for a long time. Then, heart failure often evolves in episodes during which signs of hydrosodic retention or peripheral hypoperfusion appear, interspersed with phases of relative stability. These episodes are often favored by aggravating factors that must be systematically investigated.

## 2. Criteria for the diagnosis of CI (Framingham):[1]

- **Major criteria:**

- paroxysmal nocturnal dyspnea

- jugular turgor

- crackling rales

- radiological cardiomegaly

-   acute pulmonary oedema

-   third heart sound (B3)

-   increased central venous pressure (> 16 cm of water in the right atrium)

-   circulation time greater than 25 seconds

-   hepato jugular reflux

-   pulmonary edema, visceral congestion or cardiomegaly at autopsy

-   **Minor criteria:**

-   bilateral ankle edema

-   exertional dyspnea for everyday activities

-   hepatomegaly

-   pleural effusion

-   decrease in vital capacity of more than one third of the maximum recorded value

-   tachycardia greater than 120 beats per minute (min)

-   **Other criteria:**

- weight loss > 4.5 kg in 5 days in response to treatment for heart failure

The diagnosis of heart failure requires the presence of two major criteria or one major criterion plus two minor criteria, which are accepted provided that they cannot be attributed to another condition.

The functional signs encountered in patients in decreasing order were dyspnea 100%, cough 73.78%, chest pain 49.5% and palpitations 34.95%. Dyspnea was the constant symptom found in all patients (100%) with 94 patients (91.26%) at NYHA stage IV.

Congestive heart failure is the most frequent form found in 76.70% of cases with a predominance of males. Left heart failure is observed in 20.38%. Right heart failure is the least frequent found only in 2.91%. [15]

## 3.    Heart failure with preserved left ventricular ejection fraction (LVEF) [36]

The diagnosis of heart failure with preserved left ventricular ejection fraction remains difficult. The left ventricular ejection fraction is normal and the signs and symptoms of heart failure are often nonspecific.

To improve the specificity of the diagnosis of heart failure with preserved ejection fraction, the clinical diagnosis should be supported by objective measurements of cardiac dysfunction at rest or during exercise.

The diagnosis requires that the following conditions are met:

The presence of symptoms and/or signs of heart failure

A "preserved" ejection fraction (EF) (defined as LVEF > 50%)

High NP levels (BNP 35 pg / mL and / or NT-proBNP 125 pg / mL)

Objective evidence of cardiac functional and structural alterations underlying heart failure

If there is uncertainty, a stress test or elevated left ventricular filling pressure may be necessary to confirm the diagnosis.

## II.  Cardiovascular risk factors

Hypertension, diabetes, smoking and obesity were the risk factors found in our patients with 57.28%, 8.73%, 12.62%, 5.82% respectively. The most frequent risk factor was hypertension with a male predominance (men 33% versus women 24.28%). [15]

**Table 2**: Cardiovascular risk factors and by gender. [15]

| Factors Of risk | Male | Female | Total | Percentage (%) |
|---|---|---|---|---|
| HTA | 34 | 25 | 59 | 57,28 |

| Diabetes | 6 | 3 | 9 | 8,73 |
| Tobacco | 13 | ■ | 13 | 12,62 |
| Alcohol | 3 | ■ | 3 | 2,91 |
| Obesity | 3 | 3 | 6 | 5,82 |

## III. Etiological diagnosis:[26]

The search for the cause of the heart disease is all the more important when the patient is young and can lead to the initiation of a specific treatment.

### 1. Causes of left heart failure

### 1.1 Ischemic heart disease

Ischemic heart disease, constitute, the main etiology of heart failure in 35.92% of cases with a predominance of male gender [15]

- In the acute phase of myocardial infarction (MI). Heart failure is proportional to the extent of necrosis. Rupture of the SIV or of a pillar, a rhythm disorder are aggravating factors.

- After the infarction. Sequential hypo- or akinesia, compliance disorder in the scar territory, left ventricular aneurysm, and recurrent MI are factors in left ventricular failure.

- Heart failure with a primary appearance may reveal advanced coronary artery disease (value of coronary angiography).

### 1.2 Hypertensive heart disease

- Essential or secondary.

It is the second cause of heart failure in 31.06% of cases with a predominance of the male sex. Hypertension, constitutes a real public health problem and is the main cause of heart failure in African adults [15].

### 1.3 Heart disease due to mechanical overload of the left ventricle

**Valvular heart disease:**

- **During aortic stenosis**

- Left ventricular failure is late, has a poor prognosis and requires aortic valve replacement.

- **Mitral insufficiency (MI)**

- Chronic MI:

* The volume overload creates a progressive dilation of the left ventricle. The stretching of the fibers allows the conservation of the cardiac output according to Starling's law and avoids the rise of the capillary pressure. Beyond a certain degree of stretching, adaptation is no longer possible and congestive signs appear.

- Acute mitral insufficiency (MI):

* by cord rupture or pillar dysfunction. The left ventricle (LV) does not have time to dilate

- Aside:

- functional mitral insufficiency.

- **Aortic insufficiency (AI)**

- **Left heart failure without ventricular failure**

**left: mitral dam**

- Mitral stenosis.

- Myxoma of the left atrium encasing the mitral valve.

- Mitral prosthesis thrombosis.

- **Valve prosthesis dysfunctions**

- They lead to heart failure, usually acute, due to obstruction or leakage.

**Congenital heart disease**

- Interventricular communication.

- Persistence of the ductus arteriosus.

- Coarctation of the aorta.

- Lead to left heart failure in adulthood.

**High output heart failure**

- During avitaminosis B1 (beriberi).

- Paget's disease.

- Important arteriovenous fistulas.

- Hyperthyroidism.

- Severe anemia.

- There is initially preserved left ventricular outflow, but secondary progression to low-flow heart failure.

**N.B.:** mechanical overloads are also sometimes classified according to their physiopathology:

- Pressure overload :

* aortic stenosis;

* HTA;

* aortic coarctation.

- Volume overload:

* mitral insufficiency;

* interventricular communication (IVC).

* Mixed overload (volume and pressure):

* aortic insufficiency;

* persistence of the ductus arteriosus;

* high output heart failure.

## 1.4 Cardiomyopathies by primary alteration of the cardiac muscle

**Inflammatory attack of the myocardium (myocarditis)**

- Viral: coxsackie, influenza, echovirus, HIV, hepatitis...

- Bacterial: staphylococcus, salmonella, Lyme, Q fever, diphtheria, tetanus.

- Fungal: Aspergillus, Candida.

- Parasitic: Chaggas disease, toxoplasmosis.

- Non-infectious myocarditis: collagenosis.

- Giant cell myocarditis of unknown etiology.

**Metabolic cardiomyopathy**

- Endocrinopathy: myxedema, thyrotoxicosis, acromegaly, Cushing's syndrome.

- Nutritional deficiency: B1 deficiency, kwashiorkor, selenium or carnitine deficiency.

**Toxic and hypersensitivity cardiomyopathy**

- Alcohol.

- Adriamycin, 5-FU.

- Others: emetine, Endoxan, bleomycin, cobalt, cocaine.

**Infiltrative cardiomyopathy**

- Cardiac amyloidosis.

- Hemochromatosis.

- Neoplasia, leukemia.

- Fabri's disease.

- Glycogenosis (Gaucher).

- Sarcoidosis.

**Genetic cardiomyopathies**

- Genetic mutations of different contractile proteins responsible for **hypertrophic** cardiomyopathy - muscular dystrophies: Duchenne, Becker.

- Neuromuscular disorders: Friedrich's ataxia, Noonan's syndrome.

**Endomyocardiofibrosis**

- Fibrosis and fibroelastosis of the endocardium, carcinoid.

## 1.5 Other causes

- Postpartum cardiomyopathy.

- Post-irradiation cardiomyopathy or hypothermia.

## 1.6 Idiopathic (frequent)

• By definition, cardiomyopathies (or cardiomyopathies) are primary attacks on the heart muscle (myocyte or interstitium).

• They include 4 clinico-pathological entities:

- dilated cardiomyopathy;

- hypertrophic cardiomyopathy;

- restrictive cardiomyopathy;

- arrhythmogenic dysplasia of the right ventricle (RV).

- However, a picture of dilated cardiomyopathy can also (often!) correspond to ischemic (coronary), valvular or hypertensive cardiac damage.

## 2. Causes of right CI

## 2.1 Chronic Pulmonary Heart (CPC)

**Chronic obstructive pulmonary disease**

• In the foreground are chronic bronchitis, centrilobular emphysema, asthma with continuous dyspnea, extensive bronchial dilatation (BDD); panlobular emphysema is rarely involved.

- In these diseases, right ventricular failure is late, progressive in onset, preceded by a stage of chronic "pre-capillary" pulmonary hypertension; it is often precipitated or aggravated by bronchopulmonary superinfection.

## 2.2 Restrictive lung diseases

- They are complicated very late by VDI.

- Thoracic deformities: kyphoscoliosis.

- Parietal, pleural or pulmonary sequelae after trauma, thoracic surgery, or in case of skeletal deformity: kyphoscoliosis, extensive thoracoplasties.

- It is often associated with post-smoking COPD (mixed syndrome).

- Pickwick's syndrome.

- Sequelae of neuromuscular diseases: polio, ALS, myasthenia.

## 2.3 Pulmonary disorders due to alveolocapillary diffusion anomalies

- Pulmonary fibrosis: either primary or secondary to sarcoidosis, collagenosis, histiocytosis X, pneumoconiosis.

## 2.4 Vascular causes

- Chronic post-embolic pulmonary heart (repeated embolisms).

- Chronic pulmonary heart post bilharzia.

- Primary pulmonary arterial hypertension (PAH), which is rare and must remain a diagnosis of elimination.

## 2.5 Heart disease

### Left ventricular failure (LVF)

- Most common cause of IVD (>80%).

- All causes of GVI can cause IVD, resulting in a picture of congestive heart failure. In the course of infarction, DVI leads to a search for extension to the VD, IVC, or pulmonary embolism.

- IVD reduces the importance of pulmonary manifestations, but marks a serious evolutionary turning point, testifying to the advanced nature of the cardiopathy.

**Advanced mitral stenosis with pre-capillary PAH**

**Isolated tricuspid insufficiencies: endocarditis, carcinoids**

**2.6  Acute right ventricular failure (RVF)**

- Pulmonary embolism

- Asthmatic malaise.

- Suffocating pneumothorax

- Acute bilateral lung disease

- Massive atelectasis

The table summarizes the causes of heart failure in a prospective study in Niger **[15]**

**Table 3:** Most common causes of heart failure [15]

| Etiologies | Male | Female | Total | Percentage(%) |
|---|---|---|---|---|
| **Ischemic heart disease** | 27 | 10 | 37 | 35,92 |
| **Hypertensive heart disease** | 22 | 10 | 32 | 31,06 |
| **Rheumatic heart disease** | 3 | 9 | 12 | 11,65 |
| **Hypertrophic CM** | 2 | 1 | 3 | 2,91 |
| **CMPP** | - | 8 | 8 | 7,76 |
| **Cardiothyreosis** | - | 1 | 1 | 0,97 |
| **Rhythmic heart disease** | - | 1 | 1 | 0,97 |
| **CPC** | 2 | 2 | 4 | 3,88 |
| **Pericarditis** | 2 | 2 | 4 | 3,88 |
| **Endocarditis** | 1 | - | 1 | 0,97 |

# DECOMPENSATION FACTORS: [26, 37, 38, 39, 40]

Except in the most extreme cases, generally observed in quite clearly defined situations such as amyloidosis, diabetes or severe primary hypertrophic heart disease, the telediastolic pressure is only moderately increased, explaining the paucity of symptoms at rest or during moderate efforts. It is therefore not surprising to find in the vast majority of cases, triggering factors at the origin of an increase in left ventricular end-diastolic pressure: (tachycardia, atrial fibrillation, acute volume overload, anemia). Often the triggering factors act through multiple mechanisms. Thus an ischemic attack reduces contractility, prolongs relaxation, reduces the real and apparent distensibility of the left ventricle. A hypertensive surge prolongs relaxation and may alter contractility by ischemia of the subendocardial areas and increased afterload. Tachycardia reduces filling time, may lead to subendocardial ischemia, and may be accompanied by loss of atrial contribution to filling in atrial fibrillation.

- Any infection: broncho-pulmonary, endocarditis... ;

- Salt-free diet deviation;

- Treatment: interruption, error (negative inotropic), adverse effect, hydrosodic overload, transfusion;

- Rhythm disorders (complete arrhythmia by atrial fibrillation, bradycardia, ventricular tachycardia);

- Surgical procedure, pulmonary embolism;

- Hyperflow states: anemia, pregnancy, hyperthyroidism;

- Evolution of the causative disease: hypertensive relapse, recurrence of myocardial infarction, aggravation of valvular disease.

# TREATMENT OF HEART FAILURE

Only the curative treatment of a possible etiology (valvulopathy, ischemia, hypertension...) allows to stabilize or even to regress the heart failure. All other treatments are only palliative measures to stabilize and delay the evolution of heart failure. [26]

## I.  Treatment goals [6,7]

The goals of treatment in patients with heart failure are:

Improve patient life expectancy and quality of life

Reduction in the number and duration of hospitalizations

Reduction of mortality

Slowing down the progression of the disease

Three steps are mandatory: [6]

- treatment of the cause of the CI whenever possible;

- treatment of the causes of decompensation of cardiac disease ;

- monitoring the status of congestive heart failure.

For this third step, the following objectives can be set:

- reduce the workload of the heart, preload and afterload ;

- improve myocardial contractility;

- control of hydrosodic retention.

## II.  General measures

Hygienic-dietary measures remain important and must be adapted to the patient's age and physical condition, eating habits and lifestyle. [41, 42]

They include:

❖ **the de-sodified diet** (an intake of 2 to 3 g/d of sodium chloride is tolerated). The

Strict de-sodium diet (2 g/d of sodium) is reserved for heart failure attacks.

❖ **monitoring of fluid intake**. A water restriction of 1.5 to 2 liters is recommended.

❖ **Moderate consumption of alcoholic beverages** is acceptable, prohibited if alcoholic cardiomyopathy is suspected.

❖ **weight control**

It is advisable for overweight heart failure patients to lose weight, as obesity increases the work of the left ventricle.

Clinical or subclinical malnutrition exists in about 50% of patients with severe heart failure. The decrease in total body fat and body mass that accompanies weight loss is called cardiac cachexia. This condition is predictive of reduced survival. **[43]**

❖ **control of cardiovascular risk factors**

Smoking should be avoided. The patient should be actively helped to quit smoking, including with nicotine replacement therapy.

Diabetes, hypertension and lipid disorders must be managed.

❖ rest is not desirable in stable chronic heart failure, whereas it is in acute heart failure or during decompensation of chronic heart failure.

Patients should be encouraged to engage in daily physical activity.

❖ **general advice:**

❖ Vaccination: Vaccination against influenza and pneumococcal infections can reduce the incidence of respiratory infections, which are themselves factors in the aggravation of CHF.

❖ Travel: high altitude or very hot and humid sites should be avoided.

❖ Drugs to avoid or use with caution are

o  non-steroidal anti-inflammatory drugs

o  class 1 anti-arrhythmics

o calcium channel blockers (verapamil, diltiazem, first generation dihydropyridines)

o Tricyclic antidepressants and lithium

corticosteroids.

❖  think about a possible professional reclassification

❖  cardiovascular rehabilitation = exercise rehabilitation

## III. Treatment of heart failure with impaired left ventricular ejection fraction:[36]

**Recommended treatments for all symptomatic patients**

**1.  Angiotensin-converting enzyme (ACE) inhibitors**

ACE inhibitors have been shown to reduce mortality and morbidity and are recommended unless contraindicated or intolerant in all symptomatic patients. ACE inhibitors should be used at the maximum tolerated dose to achieve adequate inhibition of the renin-angiotensin-aldosterone system (RAAS). There is evidence that in clinical practice, the majority of patients receive suboptimal doses of ACEIs. They are also recommended in patients with asymptomatic left ventricular systolic dysfunction to reduce the risk of developing symptomatic heart failure, hospitalization and death.

The molecules used are represented in the table

**Table 4**: ACEI dosing

| Molecules / IECA | Initial dose | Maximum dose |
|---|---|---|
| **Captopril:**<br><br>**LOPRIL®** CAPTOLANE ® Cp 25 and 50 mg | 6.12 mg three times /day | 50 mg three times a day |
| **Enalapril:** | 2.5 mg twice a day | 20 mg twice a day |

| | | |
|---|---|---|
| **RENITEC®** Cp 5 and 20 mg | | |
| **Lisinopril**<br><br>PRINIVIL ® **Cp 20 mg** | 5 mg taken once a day | 35 mg taken once a day |
| **Ramipril:**<br><br>**TRIATEC®** 1.25; 2.5; 5 and 10 mg | 2.5 mg taken once a day | 10 mg taken once a day |
| **Trandolapril**<br><br>GOPTEN ® **gel 0.5 mg** | 0.5 mg taken once a day | 4 mg taken once a day |
| **Perindopril:**<br><br>COVERSYL® **Cp** 4 and 8 mg | 4 mg taken once a day | 8 mg taken once a day |

- ACE inhibitors are now the reference treatment for heart failure and should be used as early as NYHA stage I.

- Side effects and contraindications:

• arterial hypotension

• dry cough

• hyperkalemia

• leukopenia, thrombocytopenia

• rash,

• angioneurotic edema

• teratogenic effect, especially in the second and third trimester renal failure

## 2. Beta-blockers

Beta-blockers reduce mortality and morbidity in symptomatic heart failure patients with impaired left ventricular ejection fraction. Beta-blockers and ACE inhibitors are complementary, and can be started together as soon as the diagnosis is established. There is no evidence to support the initiation of beta-blocker therapy before the initiation of an ACE inhibitor. Beta-blockers should be initiated in clinically stable patients at a low dose and gradually increased to the maximum tolerated dose.

Beta-blockers should be used for heart rate control in patients with atrial fibrillation, especially in those with a high heart rate.

Beta-blockers are recommended in patients with a history of myocardial infarction and asymptomatic left ventricular systolic dysfunction.

- **Usable drugs: [7]**

Four (4) beta-blockers have marketing authorization in heart failure and are summarized in the table:

**Table 5**: Beta-blocker dosing

| Molecules / Beta-blockers | Initial dose | Maximum dose |
|---|---|---|
| **Bisoprolol:** <br><br> CARDENSIEL® Cp 1,25 ; 2,5 and 5mg, DETENSIEL ® Cp 10mg | 1.25 mg taken once a day | 10 mg taken once a day |
| **Carvedilol:** <br><br> KREDEX ® Cp 6,25; 12,50 and 25mg, | 3.125 mg twice a day | 25 mg twice a day |
| **Metoprolol:** <br><br> SELOKEN®, LOPRESSOR® 100 and 200 mg. | 25 mg taken once a day | 200 mg taken once a day |
| **Nevibolol:** <br><br> TEMERIT ® Cp 5mg and 10mg, | 1.25 mg taken once a day | 10 mg taken once a day |

- **Contraindications**

They are common to all beta-blockers:

- acute heart failure;

- cardiogenic shock;

- Unfitted 2nd and 3rd degree AVB;

- sino-auricular block;

- bradycardia < 50/min prior to initiation of therapy ;

- arterial hypotension; (systolic < 90 mm Hg);

- Raynaud's syndrome and peripheral arterial disorders ;

- severe asthma or COPD;

- untreated pheochromocytoma ;

- metabolic acidosis;

- allergy to bisoprolol.

- **Method of administration**

Initiation of beta-blocker therapy should be done at a distance from any acute episode (within the previous six weeks);

The initial dosage is low;

Beta-blocker doses are increased in increments of one week to 15 days, under strict supervision. In case of intolerance, do not stop abruptly but reduce the dosage to the previous level.

**3.   Mineralocorticoid/aldosterone receptor antagonists (MRAs) [36]**

MRAs (spironolactone and eplerenone) block aldosterone receptors and, with varying degrees of affinity, other steroid hormone receptors (e.g. corticosteroids, androgens). Spironolactone or eplerenone is recommended in all symptomatic patients (despite treatment with ACE inhibitors and beta-blockers) with LVEF <35%, to reduce mortality and hospitalization.

Precautions should be taken when using MRAs in patients with renal impairment. Regular monitoring of serum potassium and renal function should be performed according to clinical status.

❖ **Usable Medications**

- Indicated at low dose in combination with ACEI + BB + ANSE diuretic

**Table 6**: Dosage of antialdosterones

| Molecules | Initial dose | Maximum dose |
|---|---|---|
| **Spironolactone**<br>ALDACTONE ® Cp 50 and 75 mg | 25 mg taken once a day | 75 mg taken once a day |
| **Eplerenone**<br>INSPRA 25 and 50 mg | 25 mg taken once a day | 50 mg taken once a day |
| **Spironolactone + Thiazide**<br>ALDACTIAZIDE® Cp 25 mg and 50 mg, | 25 mg taken once / jour | 50 mg taken once / jour |

- **Contraindications**:

- two are essential: renal insufficiency and hyperkalemia.

- obstruction of the urinary tract

- severe hepatic insufficiency

## 4. Diuretics

- **Diuretics of ANSE**

Diuretics are recommended to reduce congestive signs and symptoms, but their effects on mortality and morbidity have not been demonstrated.

The goal of diuretic therapy is to achieve and maintain euvolemia with the lowest possible dose. The dose of diuretic should be adjusted according to individual needs over time. In selected asymptomatic euvolemic/hypovolemic patients, the use of diuretic medication could be discontinued (temporarily). **[36]**

- **Usable drugs**

- **Furosemide (LASILIX ®): 20, 40, or 60 and 500 mg tablets**

**20 and 250 mg ampoules**

Usual dosage: 20 to 60 mg/24 h (much higher doses in case of edema of the lower limbs or renal insufficiency), 2 Cp per day maximum if 500 mg tablet.

- **Bumetanide (BURINEX®): 1 and 5 mg tablets**

**0.5, 2 and 5 mg ampoules**

- dosage 1 to 3 tablets per day, 1 mg BURINEX = 40 mg LASILIX

- oppose the tubular reabsorption of sodium Na+.

- increase glomerular blood flow.

- promote vasodilatation of the venous capacitance system.

- have a dose-response role, which allows for increased doses in cases of renal failure and severe abortion.

- by injection, remain the emergency treatment of OAP.

- **Counter indications**:

- allergies to sulphonamides

- obstruction of the urinary tract

- extra-cellular dehydration, hypovolemia

- uncorrected fluid and electrolyte disorders (hyponatremia below 130 mmol/l, hypokalemia)

- pregnancy (bumetamide) and lactation

- severe hepatic encephalopathy or cirrhosis

- **Known side effects**: hypokalemia, hyponatremia, hypochloremia, extracellular dehydration, orthostatic hypotension, functional renal failure). **[7, 26]**

- **Thiazide diuretics**

- **Usable drugs**

- Clopamide (BRINADIX ®) Cp 20 mg, ^ to 3 Cp per day

- Hydrochlorothiazide (ESIDREX ®) Cp 25 mg, 1 to 4 Cp per day

- Chlortalidone (HYGROTON ®) Cp 25 mg, 1 to 2 mg per day

- Indapamide (FLUDEX ®) Cp 2.5 mg, 1 Cp per day

- **Contraindications**:

- allergies to sulphonamides

- obstruction of the urinary tract

- renal insufficiency (creatinine > 200 mmol/l or > 25 mg)

- uncorrected hydro-electrolytic disorders.

They are usually combined with potassium-sparing diuretics.

## 5. Angiotensin II type I receptor blockers

ARBs are recommended only as an alternative in patients with contraindication or intolerance to ACE inhibitors. Candesartan has been shown to reduce cardiovascular mortality. The combination of ARB II and ACE inhibitors is not recommended. [**36**]. They share the same contraindications as ACE inhibitors.

**Table 7**: ARB II dosing

| Molecules | Initial dose | Maximum dose |
|---|---|---|
| Candesartan<br><br>ATACAND 4, 8 and 16 mg | 4 mg taken once a day | 32 mg taken once a day |
| Valasartan<br><br>TAREG 40, 80 and 160 mg | 40 mg twice a day | 160 mg twice a day |
| Losartan<br><br>COZAAR 50, 100 and 150 mg | 50 mg taken once a day | 150 mg taken once a day |

## 6. Vasodilators in heart failure

- **Vasodilators with predominantly venous action**

- **Nitrate derivatives:[7, 44]**

By reducing preload, they improve signs of pulmonary congestion, without directly altering myocardial function.

They can be used in all forms of left ventricular failure unless contraindicated.

- **By sublingual route** (short action, a few minutes):

o **Trinitrine: NATISPRAY FORT®**, spray at 0.30 mg per puff, one puff under the tongue.

o **Isosorbite Dinitrate RISORDAN ®** Cp 5 mg to be melted under the tongue.

- **By parenteral route,**

o **LENITRAL®** inj with electric          syringe

o **RISORDAN®** inj

- **Oral**:

o RISORDAN **LP®** 20, 20          mg1Cp   twice daily

o RISORDAN **LP®** 40, 40          mg1Cp   twice daily

o Molsidomine : CORVASAL ® 2 and 4 mg 1 Cp twice a day

- **Contraindications**:

• apart from a blood pressure that is too low for the use of the venous route, there are no major contraindications to the use of nitrates, apart from their association with sildenafil (viagra®)

• however, their use with other vasodilators or diuretics should be cautious in the elderly because of the risk of hypotension.

• right ventricular infarction

• Side effects:

• headaches

• orthostatic hypotension

• **Pure arterial vasodilators**

They are currently little used.

By decreasing afterload, they decrease cardiac work and improve ventricular ejection. Low output heart failure with low capillary pressure is their best indication.

## 7.    Inhibitor of the if channel [36].

Ivabradine slows the heart rate through inhibition of the if channel of the sinus node and therefore should only be used in patients in sinus rhythm. Ivabradine reduces mortality and hospitalization for decompensation in symptomatic patients with LVEF <35%, in sinus rhythm and with a heart rate >70 beats per minute who had been hospitalized for heart failure in the previous 12 months, receiving beta-blocker therapy (maximum tolerated dose), ACEI (or ARB) and ARM.

Ivabradine: **PROCORALAN 5 mg and 7.5 mg film-coated tablet**

The usual recommended starting dose is **5 mg of ivabradine twice daily.**

**After two weeks of treatment, the dose can be :**

*S* **increased** to 7.5 mg twice daily if resting heart rate remains

persistently above 60 beats per minute.

*S* **or reduced** to 2.5 mg twice a day (i.e., half a 5 mg tablet 2

Once a day) if the resting heart rate is persistently below 50 beats per minute or if symptoms related to bradycardia such as dizziness, fatigue or hypotension occur.

If the heart rate is between 50 and 60 beats per minute, the dosage of 5 mg twice daily can be maintained.

## 8.    Digitalisers and positive inotropes

All tonicardiacs act by increasing the level of intracellular calcium available in systole for contraction.

Digoxin may only be recommended for the treatment of atrial fibrillation patients with rapid ventricular rate when other therapeutic options cannot be pursued (contraindication to beta-blockers) [36]

Digoxin may be considered in symptomatic patients in sinus rhythm to reduce the risk of hospitalization (all causes).

**Digitalisms [44]**

**- Digoxin:**

**o DIGOXINE ® Cp 0.25 mg 1cp/d every day**

**IV ampoule of 0.05 mg** 1 ampoule in IVL then ^ ampoule to 1 ampoule to renew if needed.

By inhibiting the membrane sodium Na+/K+ ATPase pump, they increase intracellular sodium and calcium levels.

Digitalis are unquestionably useful in left ventricular failure accompanied by rapid atrial fibrillation. They are no longer indicated in the absence of atrial fibrillation. There is a narrow margin between therapeutic and toxic doses, especially in elderly patients or those with advanced myocardial failure. This margin requires:

• **Prescription and monitoring rules:**

• no loading dose;

• monitoring of congestive signs, heart rate, blood ionogram;

• knowledge of drug interferences (quinidine...);

• precautions of use, even abstention in case of renal insufficiency (for digoxin with renal elimination) or hepatic insufficiency (for digitoxin withdrawn from the market with hepatobiliary elimination).

• reduction of doses in the elderly (generally by half).

**- Knowledge of situations favouring intoxication:** hypokalemia, hypoxia, acidosis, hypercalcemia.

**- Clinical monitoring for signs of intoxication:** nausea, vomiting, severe sinus bradycardia, rhythm disturbances (ASD, ESV), atrioventricular conduction disorders.

- **Knowledge of contraindications:**

• ventricular rhythm disorders (ESV, VT).

• BAV, sino-auricular block, Wolff-Parkinson-White.

• CMO, RA tight.

• advanced myocardial failure (risk of ineffectiveness at usual doses).

• recent electric shocks.

• **Use of serum digitalis assays:**

J after reaching steady state, i.e. 6 to 10 days for digoxin.

J in case of suspected intoxication.

J to learn about medication adherence.

J after modification of dosage.

• **Knowledge of the electrical signs of myocardial impregnation by digitalis :**

• appearance of a digital cup (inferior and concave upward shift of the ST segment).

• QT shortening.

• **Digitalis intoxication**

• Extra Cardiac Signs:

o **digestive signs**: anorexia, nausea, vomiting, abdominal pain, transit disorders.

o **Ocular signs**: yellow-green dyschromatopsia with light flashes, pathognomonic sign.

o **neurological signs**: headaches, confusion, dizziness, convulsions. psychiatric disorders are common in the elderly. however, digitalis intoxication is not a cause of coma.

• Sines and cardiac complications:

o   bradycardia

o   atrial tachycardia

o   ventricular extrasystole, ventricular tachycardia, fibrillation

ventricular

o   cardiogenic shock

o   asystole

## 9. Positive inotropic agents

- **Sympathomimetics**

Amines that can be used by the IV route with an electric syringe pump: Dobutamine: DOBUTREX ® 5 to 20µg/kg/mn, Dopamine: 20 to 30µg/kg/mn.

They are used in the treatment of the majority of acute cardiac failures in the resuscitation setting (cardiogenic shock), under control of pulmonary capillary pressure. They act by stimulating membrane adenylcyclase, which converts adenosine triphosphate (ATP) into cyclic adenosine monophosphate (AMP).

- **Phosphodiesterase inhibitors (IV only) (Iconor, Corotrope, Perfane)**

They prevent cAMP degradation by increasing intracellular calcium entry and myocardial relaxation rate. They have an associated arterial vasodilator effect.

Their undesirable effects (thrombocytopenia) prevent prolonged per os use. Only parenteral use in a hospital setting is possible, either briefly or discontinuously, in cases of refractory heart failure.

Their indication is more and more discussed.

- **Levosimendan**

The first drug in a new class, it acts by increasing the sensitivity of the contractile apparatus of myocytes to calcium. It is currently being evaluated but looks promising.

**IV. Treatment of heart failure with preserved left ventricular ejection fraction. [36]**

No treatment has yet been convincingly shown to reduce morbidity or mortality in preserved FECG IC patients. However, since these patients are often elderly and highly symptomatic, and often with poor quality of life, an important goal of treatment may be to relieve symptoms and improve quality of life.

Diuretics usually improve congestion, if present, thereby ameliorating the symptoms and signs of heart failure. There is no evidence on the effectiveness of beta-blockers and mineralocorticoid receptor antagonists.

**V. Other treatments**

**1. Anticoagulant treatment**

Necessary in cases of atrial fibrillation, significant dilatation of the heart chambers with low flow or intracavitary thrombus.

**2. Antiarrhythmic treatment:[45]**

- Amiodarone (CORDARONE ®) Cp 200 mg, Ampoule 150 mg

o   if atrial fibrillation or flutter

o   if ventricular tachycardia

- Class I and IV anti-arrhythmics are contraindicated. [7]

**3. Multi-site pacing: ventricular resynchronization [7, 26]**

- Multisite pacing is a technique under development; its objective is to resynchronize the two ventricles (especially in cases of very large left bundle branch block) and to optimize the atrioventricular delay. In some patients, multisite pacing allows an improvement of the systolic performance of the left ventricle.

- In practice, several leads are inserted (right ventricle, left ventricle through the coronary sinus and right atrium). The pacemaker is programmed to activate both ventricles together.

- Indication: NYHA stage III-IV patients under optimal medical treatment with dilated LV and LVEF less than or equal to 35%, in sinus rhythm and a wide QRS greater than or equal to 120 milliseconds.

## 4. Automatic implantable defibrillator

Implantable automatic defibrillator placement is considered in patients with either recovered sudden death or severe ventricular rhythm disorders resistant to maximal antiarrhythmic therapy. The decision to implant is made on a case-by-case basis.

## 5. Treatment of last resort

### Circulatory assistance

Different systems have been developed:

- **diastolic counterpulsation by intra-aortic balloon**;

- **ventricular assist pump** ;

- **total artificial heart**.

Their indication is reserved for refractory heart failure when there is a prospect of treatment (transplantation) or recovery (myocarditis, for example).

### Heart transplantation

### Indications:

- stage III or IV heart failure with very low maximal oxygen consumption (VO2), after failure of conventional treatments.

### Contraindications:

- age over 60 or 65 years old.

- neoplasia or severe systemic disease.

- precapillary pulmonary hypertension (PAH)

- insulin-dependent diabetes.

- active infection (hepatitis, HIV in particular).

- hepatic or renal dysfunction.

- severe arterial damage.

- psychosocial condition incompatible with long-term care.

**Complications:**

- acute, subacute, chronic rejection often

- renal failure.

- neoplasia.

- especially currently, immunological coronary artery disease of the graft, after a few years, not very accessible to treatment.

**Survival**

- 80% at one year.

- 70% at five years.

- 30% at ten years.

**Cardiomyoplasty**

- Surgical technique that consists of rolling up a portion of the longus dorsi muscle and stimulating it with a pacemaker that is synchronized with the heart rate.

- Advantages: no immunosuppressive treatment.

- But the results are rather disappointing, especially if the heart failure is very advanced.

# FOLLOW-UP OF THE PATIENT WITH HEART FAILURE: [7]

## I. Objectives

- Identify potentially reversible aggravating factors

- Identify concomitant pathologies that may influence CI and its treatment.

- Ensure that the patient and his or her family have understood the dietary measures and the treatment.

- Ensure that care is appropriate.

## II. Professionals involved

- Cardiologist

- Attending physician

- Nurse

- Dietician if obese

- Specialized addiction center: alcohol withdrawal

- Multidisciplinary care

## III. Follow-up

### 1. Clinic

**Interrogation**

- Activities of Daily Living;

- Weight, diet and salt intake;

- Search for depression, cognitive disorders.

**Clinical examination**

- Heart rate, blood pressure, signs of fluid retention.

**Periodicity of consultations**

- If heart failure is unstable: close consultations++.

- At each level during the drug titration phase

- In the days following a change

- If symptoms persist: once a month

- If balanced: every 6 months

## 2. Complementary examinations necessary for follow-up

**Biology**

- Natremia, kalemia and creatinemia every 6 months or in case of intercurrent events after any significant therapeutic change.

- Depending on the initial context

- TSH, INR if anticoagulant treatment.

**ECG**: at least every 6 months

**Chest X-ray**: in case of warning signs

**Transthoracic Echocardiography**:

- in case of clinical change

- if you are undergoing treatment that may affect cardiac function

- at least every 3 years for patients who remain stable.

## PREVENTIVE OF CARDOIC INSUFFICIENCY:[7]

The prevention of heart failure is based on the suppression or control of cardiovascular diseases responsible for the failure of the heart pump. It is a public health approach that takes into account the prevalence of pathologies responsible for heart failure. Therefore, it is necessary :

- Correctly treat strep throat and rheumatic fever, which are among the leading causes of valvulopathy in underdeveloped countries;

- Treating valve disease before the onset of irreversible left ventricular dysfunction;

- Correcting congenital heart disease;

- Combat high blood pressure and/or coronary heart disease by reducing other risk factors such as smoking, diabetes, obesity, dyslipidemia;

- Eliminate or limit medications and other cardiotoxic substances (alcohol, anticancer drugs, tricyclic antidepressants)

- Eliminate the triggers of a heart failure attack (anemia, bronchopulmonary infections, hyperthyroidism,)

- Influenza and pneumococcal vaccinations

# CONCLUSION

Heart failure is a frequent and serious condition. Nevertheless, the important progress made in the diagnostic and therapeutic management of these patients has gradually allowed a significant change in the clinical physiognomy of this condition. It is currently rare to encounter patients with refractory congestive heart failure.

Currently, the heart failure patient is often an ambulatory patient, limited in his physical activity, who is hospitalized from time to time during a decompensation.

The morbidity and mortality of this disease have decreased significantly, so that we are gradually witnessing the aging of this population.

Heart failure in the elderly is a growing public health problem. Given the aging of the population, its incidence is constantly increasing.

It is a syndrome with multiple etiologies that presents certain particularities in this vulnerable segment of the population. **[46, 47]**

In the West, its prevalence is known **[47,48], but** this is not the case in sub-Saharan Africa where only hospital data are available **[49].**

# Bibliography


1. **Pousset F, Isnard R, Komjda M.** Heart failure: epidemiological, clinical and prognostic aspects. EMC. 2003- Editions Scientifiques et Médicales. Elsevier SAS, Paris. Cardiologue, 11-03G-20, 2003;2875:1171- 1186.

2. **Mahamadou BI.** Heart failure in HNN: epidemiological, clinical, paraclinical and therapeutic aspects. Thesis Méd Univ. Niamey, 200 n°1350.

3. **Delahaye F, G-de-Gevigney.** adult congestive heart failure: pathophysiology, pathophysiological forms, diagnosis and treatment; Impact internat, cardiology 2002;230:111-120.

4. **Limossin F.** Psychological aspects in heart failure. EMC (Elsevier SAS), Cardiology 11-036-G-60, 2003; 2875:1142-1158.

5. **SAR Antoine.** l"insuffisance cardiaque aiguë : pronostic, stratification des risques dans la prise en charge initiale, Thèse de médecine 2009 ; Université PARIS DIDEROT - Paris 7.

6. **Delahaye F, Juillière Y.** Insufficiency cardiaque : physiopathologie, formes physiopathologiques, clinique et traitement, Cardiologie pour le praticien, MASSON 3° édition ; 540:133-152.

7. **BESSE B, LELLOUCHE N.** Diseases and major syndromes: chronic heart failure in adults, Cardiology and Vascular Diseases, New Edition 2008;629:317-344.

8. **Ponikowski P, Adriaan AV, Stefan DA al.** ESC Guidelines for the diagnosis and treatment of acute and chronic heart failure. Eur. Heart J. 2016;128:10-85.

9. **Ballarabé I M.** Heart failure in HNN: epidemiological, clinical, paraclinical and therapeutic aspects. Thesis Méd n°1350, 2000; Univ. Niamey/Niger.

10. **Cowie MR, Moster A, Wood DA et al.** The epidemiology of heart failure. Eur. Heart J. 1997;18(2):208-25.

11. **Dickstein K, Januzzi JL, Camargo CA et al.** ESC Guidelines for the diagnosis and treatment of acute and chronic heart failure: the Task Force for the Diagnosis and

Treatment of Acute and Chronic Heart Failure 2008 of the European Society of Cardiology. Developed in collaboration with the Heart Failure Association of the ESC (HFA) and endorsed by the European Society of Intensive Care Medicine (ESICM). Eur. Heart J. 2008; 29(19):2388-442. 120.

12.  **Cullough PA, Phibin EF, Polanczyk CA, et al.** Confirmation of a heart failure epidemic: findings from the Resource Utilization Among Congestive Heart Failure (REACH) study. J. Am. Coll Cardiol 2002;39(1):60-9.

13.  **Stewart S, MacIntyre K, Macleod MC et al.** Trends in hospitalization for heart failure in Scotland, 1990-1996. An epidemic that has reached its peak? Eur. Heart J. 2001;22(3):209-17.

14.  **Menta IA.** Cardiovascular pathology of the elderly: socio demography, epidemiology, clinic, treatment, evolution (491 cases). Univ Bamako; Thesis Med. 1999; n°

15.  **Maliki AM, Harouna B, Harouna H et al.** Adult heart failure: A study of 130 hospital cases at the cardiology pole of the national hospital of Niamey, Niger . *Jaccr Africa 2018* ;2(1):139-145.

16.  **Hunt SA, Abraham WT, Chin MH, et al.** focused update incorporated into the ACC/AHA 2005 Guidelines for the Diagnosis and Management of Heart Failure in Adults: a report of the American College of Cardiology Foundation/American Heart Association Task Force on Practice Guidelines: developed in collaboration with the International Society for Heart and Lung Transplantation. Circulation, 2009;**119**(14):391-479.

17.  **Deedwania PC**. The key to unraveling the mystery of mortality in

heart failure: an integrated approach. Circulation, 2003;**107**(13):1719-21.

18.  **Rich MW**. Epidemiology, pathophysiology, and etiology of congestive heart failure in older adults. J. Am. Geriatr. Soc. 1997;**45**(8):968-74.

19.  **Delahaye F, Mercusot A, Sediq-Sarwari R.** Epidemiology of heart failure in Europe: epidemic of the 21 st century? mt cardio. 2006:*2(*1):62-72

20.  **Cowie MR, Mosterd A, Wood DA et al.** The epidemiology of heart failure. Eur. Heart J. 1997;18(2):208-25.

21.  **Ho KK, Pinsky JL, Kannel WB, et al.** The epidemiology of heart failure: the Framingham Study. J. Am. Coll. Cardiol. 1993;22:6-13.

22.  **<u>McCullough PA</u>, <u>Philbin EF</u>, <u>Spertus JA</u> et al.** Confirmation of a heart failure epidemic: findings from the Resource Utilization Among Congestive Heart Failure (REACH) study. J. Am. Coll Cardiol 2002;39(1):60-9.

23.  **Lloyd-Jones DM, Larson MG, Leip EP, et al**. Lifetime risk for developing congestive heart failure: the Framingham Heart Study. Circulation, 2002; **106**(24):3068-72.121

24.  **Lloyd-Jones D, <u>Adams R, Carnethon M</u> et al**. Heart disease and stroke statistics; update: a report from the American Heart Association Statistics Committee and Stroke Statistics Subcommittee. Circulation, 2009;**19**(3):21-181.

25.  **Cowie MR, Wood DA, Coats AJ et al**. Incidence and ctiology of heart failure; a population-based study. Eur. Heart J. 1999;**20**(6):421-8

26.  **Charles - Edouard LUYT.** Heart failure in adults HIPPOCRATE Collection, Servier Cardiology, 2003-2005;11-250.

27.  **ARONOW W S, AHIN C, KRONZON I** Normal left ventricular ejection fraction in older persons with congestive heart failure. Chest. 1998;113:867-9.

28.  **CARUANA L, PETRIE M, DOVIE A, et al.** Do patients with suspect heart failure and normal systolic function suffer from (diastolic heart failure), of from misdiagnosis. A prospective study. Br. Med. J. 2000;321:215-19.

29.  **COHEN SOLAL A**. Left ventricular diastolic dysfunction pathophysiology diagnosis and treatment Nephrol. Dis. Transplant 1998;13:3-25.

30.  **DROBINSKI G, EUGENE M.** Exploitation hémodynamique cardiovasculaire. Masson, Paris, 1982:1632p.

31.  **DELCAYRE C, SYILVESTRE JS, GAMIER A et al.** Cardiac aldosterone

production and ventricular remodeling Kidney Int. 2000;57:364-51.

**32. GROSSMAN W**. Diastolic dysfunction in congestive heart failure.

N. Engl. J. Med. 1991;325:1557-1564.

**33. CASILE JP.** left ventricular insufficiency: signs, diagnosis and treatment. Pathologies cardiovasculaires, Editions médicales heures de France; 2007:149-163

**34. Marie - Emilie, Luc Hittinger.** Adult congestive heart failure: etiologies, pathophysiology, diagnosis, evolution, treatment. Rev. Prat. Cardiologie- Pathologie vasculaire 1999:765-776.

**35. Denis Pouchain**. UFR Créteil la prise en charge du patient insuffisant cardiaque chronique. La revue exercice-Janvier/Février 2003 n°66-1.

**36. Guidelines for the diagnosis and treatment of acute and chronic heart failure.** The Task Force for the European Society of Cardiology (ESC). Eur Heart J 2016;128:14-84.

**37. LOGEART D.** Heart failure: an epidemic of the XXXth century? Euro-conference of the Pasteur Institute. La lettre du cardiologue 2000;338:6-12.

**38. THOMAS D.** Cardiology. 3rd Edition Ellipses, AUPELF/UREF. Paris, 1994;135-158.

**39. MURAKAMI T, KRAYENBUHL HP.** Influence of verapamil on diastolic left ventricular function in myocardial hypertrophy of different origin. Z. Cordial. 1987;76:82-6.

**40. LORELL BH.** Role of angiotensin AT1 and AT2 receptors in cardiac hypertrophy and disease. Am. J. Cardiol. 1999;83:448-52.

**41. ISNAR DR.** The medical treatment of the chronic heart failure patient. Ann. Cardiol. Angeiol. 2001;50:30-7.

**42. JUILLIERE Y, BERDER V,** Management of the symptomatic patient during exercise. Arch. Mal. Cœur 1998;91(11):1343-6.

**43. KONSTAM MA, PATTEN RD.** <u>Thomas I</u> et al. Effects of losartan and captopril on left ventricular volumes in elderly patients with heart failure: result oft he ELITE ventricular function substudy. Am. Heart J. 2000;139:1081-7.

**44. BESSE B, LELLOUCHE N.** Cahier therapeutique, Cardiology and Vascular Diseases, New Edition 2008;629:583-622.

**45. Cooper RS, Amoah AG, Mensah GA.** High blood pressure: the foundation for epidemic cardiovascular disease inAfrican populations. *Ethn. Dis.* 2003;3:S48-52.

**46. Emeriau JP, and Albert D**. Heart disease in the elderly. EMC Cardiology 25-802-A-10, 11-036-H-10, 1997:7.

**47. Swynghadau WB, Besse S, Heymes C, et al.** Cardiovascular system of normal elderly subjects, Cardiovascular senescence. CR. Biol. 2002;325:683-91

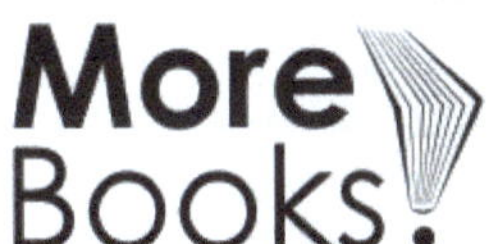

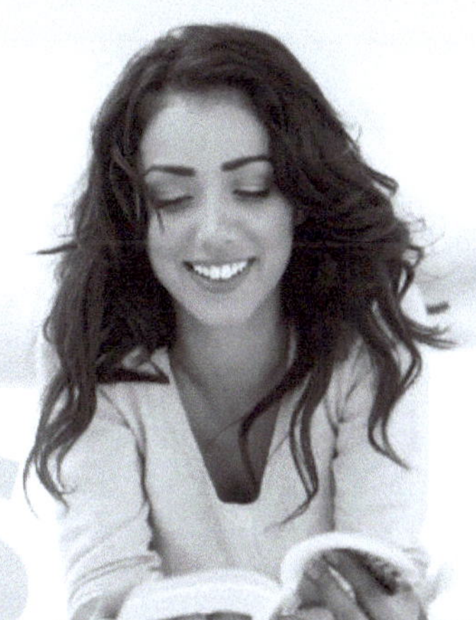

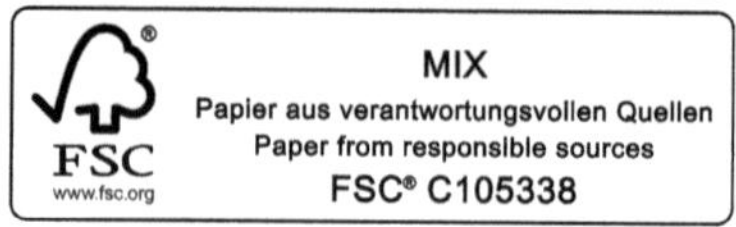

Printed by Books on Demand GmbH, Norderstedt / Germany